YOGA

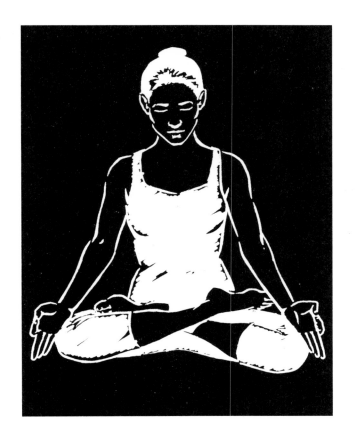

THE ESSENTIAL POSITIONS

CHARTWELL
BOOKS

Contents

Introduction   4

Standing Postures   6

Sitting Postures   30

Arm Balances   46

Back Bends   52

Forward Bends   64

Core   72

Inversions   79

Restorative   86

Types of Yoga   94

Index   96

Introduction

The word 'yoga' means union and unity, referring not only to the union of separate parts with one another, but also a unity within the complete human existence. The yoga practitioner strives to achieve a state of being where all opposites and tendencies within her or his being are reconciled into a state of unity. The Taoist symbol of yin and yang illustrates this concept – there is always a dot of black on the white, and a dot of white on the black. These opposing dots represent the balancing of opposites, which are an inevitable part of everyday life. Once we can accept the whole of our being, from our superficial tendencies down into the depths of our own individual truth, we can achieve unity with all life. To practise yoga is to honour the wholeness of which we are in each and every present moment.

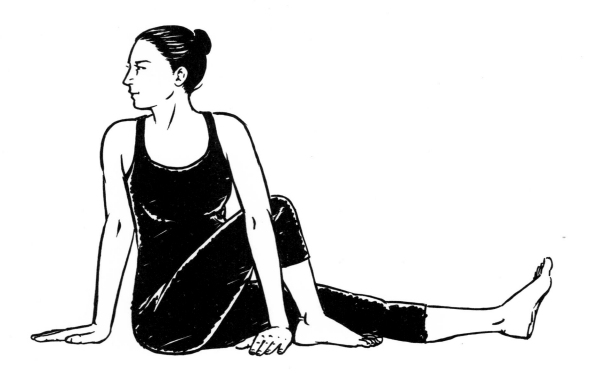

Twisted Pose I
Vakrasana

Increases mobility in the lower and upper spine and opens the hips

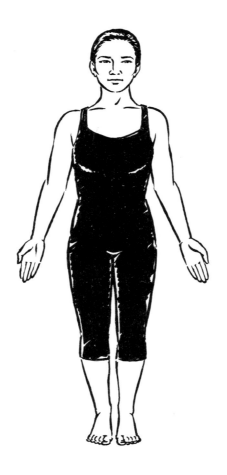

Mountain
Tadasana
Balances the whole body

Stand with the feet either hip-width apart or together. Broaden the balls of the feet and lengthen the legs in two directions up the front of the legs and down the back to the heels. Lengthen the sacrum down away from the base of the skull and lengthen upwards from the pubis to the throat. Keep the jaw parallel to the floor. Lengthen the arms in two directions up the front and down the back, with palms facing outwards at the side of the thighs.

Practice Guidelines

The postures in this book are set into sections ranging through the best sequence of a regular yoga class. You will usually start standing upright and then move on to forward bends, into back bends, arm balances, rotations or twists before doing core work, inversions and restorative work. If you want to ease gently into your pratice, begin with some of the restorative postures before starting your standing work. On some days, in the afternoon or evening, you can follow a sitting practice with restorative work, or an inversion practice followed by restorative work. Most postures are held for 5–15 breaths, depending on your level. Guidelines for this are given along with each posture.

The actions listed here apply to most of the postures and have an important impact. To get the maximum value from your yoga practice, it is important to master them. Focus on this list of postural instructions while you practice, where possible:

1. separate the ribcage from the pelvis

2. lengthen the pelvic floor from the feet

3. broaden the pelvic floor from the feet

4. engage the thighs from the feet and legs

5. lift the hip bones from the feet

6. lengthen the groin from the feet

7. soften the backs of the knees

8. soften the buttocks from the feet

9. broaden the front chest from the arms

10. broaden the back ribcage from the arms

11. broaden the top ribcage from the arms

12. lengthen the hands within the arms

13. lengthen the fingers within the arms

Standing Forward Bend
Uttanasana

Releases the lower spine

Inhale and raise the arms, keeping the shoulders relaxed, back chest open and outer shoulders gently rotated outwards. Broaden the feet fully to activate the leg muscles. As you exhale, bend the knees to release the lower spine. Bend forwards. When the chest makes contact with the thighs, grasp the legs behind the ankles. Never straighten the legs here unless the pelvis is free, the hamstrings long and the spine mobile.

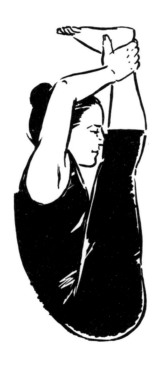

Downwards-Facing Dog
Adho Mukha Svanasana

Softens the lumbar spine and strengthens the trunk and legs

In an all-fours position on your knees, inhale. As you exhale, lengthen the buttocks upwards while keeping the knees slightly bent to protect the spine. Broaden the finger bases and feet bases to support the arms and the legs. Lengthen upwards from the heels to the buttocks. Keep the back chest open.

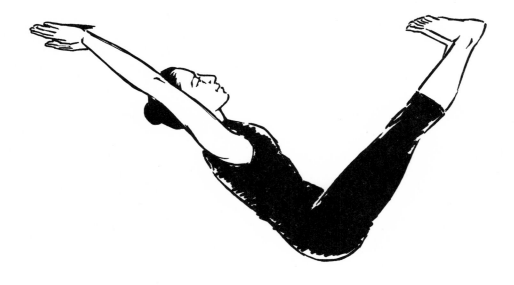

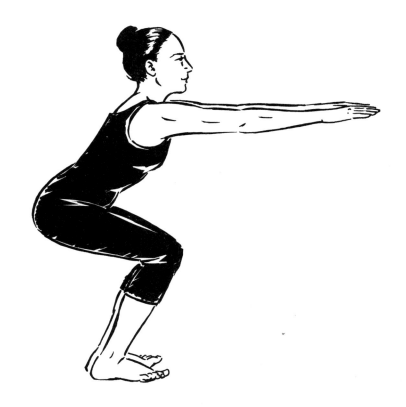

Chair Pose
Utkatasana

Strengthens the legs and spine

Standing with the feet hip-width apart, inhale and take the arms out to the side and then forwards while bending the knees deeply. Breathe freely to hold this position or exhale and come back to standing. Keep the shoulders relaxed. The hands should come no higher than the shoulder.

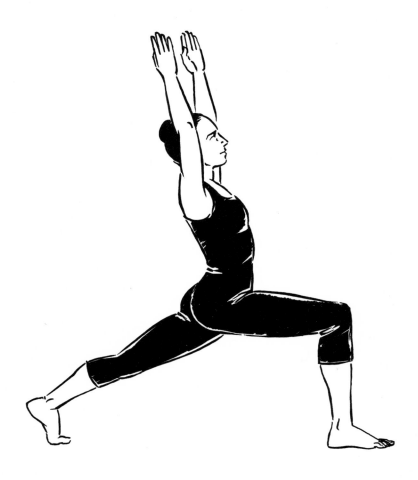

High Lunge
Utthita Ashwa Sanchalanasana

Strengthens the legs and aids balance

Stand with the right leg forwards and the left leg back, with the back heel
lifted to a 75° angle and inhale. As you exhale, bend the front right knee
to 90°. Keep the hip bones lifted and the sacrum lengthening downwards.
Breathe freely as you raise the arms upwards, keeping the shoulders
relaxed and the neck soft, then change sides and repeat.

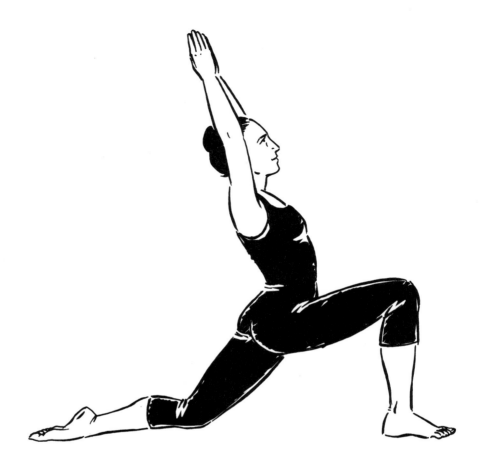

Low Lunge
Anjaneyasana

Opens the hip flexors and lengthens the spinal column

Step forwards with the right foot and bend the front right knee to 90°.
Relax the top of the left foot on the floor while pressing the left hip bone
forwards. Inhale and raise the arms upwards. As you exhale gently, look
upwards from the base of the skull, then change sides and repeat.

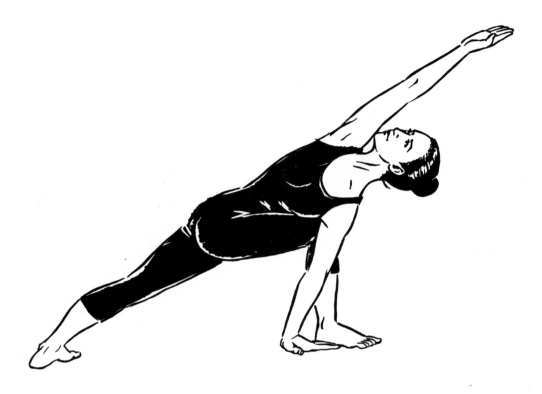

Revolved Side Lunge
Parivrtta Parsvakonasana

Maintains spinal mobility and shoulder flexibility

Step forwards with the right leg and bend the right knee to 90°. Turn the
left foot outwards by 75°. Inhale and raise both arms forwards. As you
exhale place the back of the right shoulder over the outside edge of the
right knee and set the right hand flat on the floor. Extend and lengthen the
left arm. Look gently skywards as you inhale and exhale five times, deeply
and slowly, then change sides and repeat.

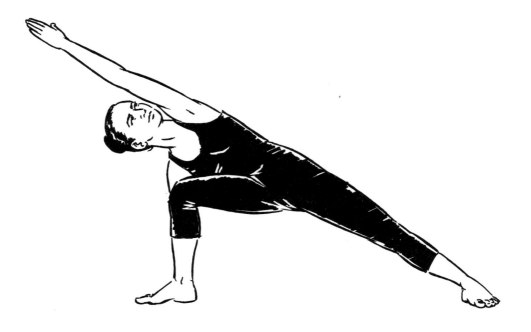

Extended Side Angle
Utthita Parsvakonasana

Lengthens and opens the waist muscles while strengthening the legs

Step forwards with the right leg. Bend the right knee to 90°. Turn the left foot outwards by 75°. Extend and lengthen the left arm and place the right hand flat on the floor outside of the right foot. Roll the ribs on your right side up to the sky, look gently upwards and inhale and exhale deeply and slowly, then change sides and repeat.

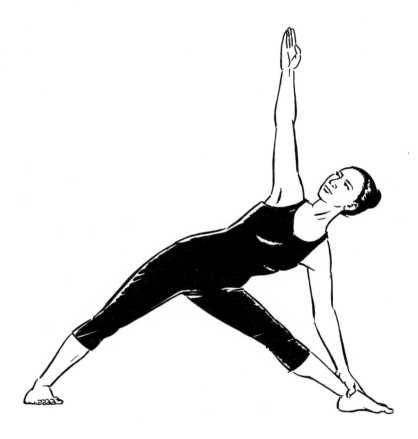

Extended Triangle
Uttihita Tikonasana
Lengthens the spine and tones the legs

Inhale and turn the left foot out to the side, keeping both legs straight but with a soft bend in the knee. Inhale and raise the arms. As you exhale, lengthen the left arm to the inside of the left leg and lengthen the right arm upwards in line with the shoulder. Inhale and exhale deeply five times, then change sides and repeat.

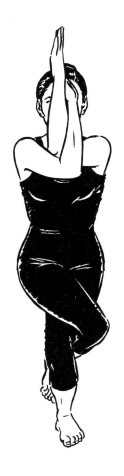

Eagle
Garudasana

Strengthens and stretches the ankles and calves and stretches the thighs, hips, shoulders and upper back

Stand upright and inhale while lifting the right knee and wrapping it around the left leg. Exhale and broaden the ball of the left foot. Inhale and open the arms. As you exhale, wrap the left forearm around the right forearm, fingers pointing straight upwards. Hold the position as you inhale and exhale deeply five times, then change sides and repeat.

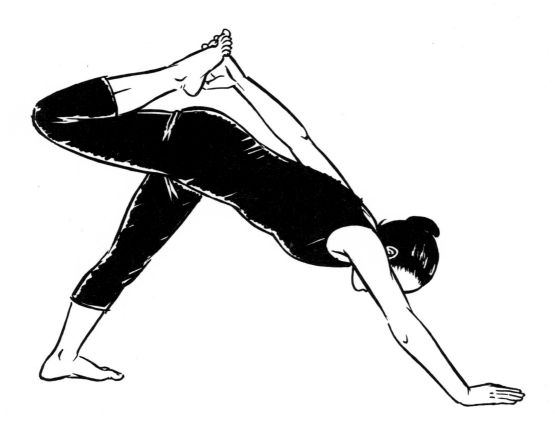

Three-Legged Dog
Eka Adhomukashasana

Lengthens the spine, opens the hips and improves leg strength and balance

From an all-fours position, inhale and, as you exhale, lengthen from the front ankles to the hip bones and down from the buttock bones to the heels to lengthen the legs to lift your trunk off the floor. Broaden the base of the fingers and the palms to support yourself. Inhale and extend the right leg up behind you. Exhale and take the left arm around and grasp the right foot. Inhale, open the front chest and exhale. Draw the right foot away from the buttocks, opening the trunk muscles and stretching the right hip while doing so. Inhale and exhale deeply five times, then change sides and repeat.

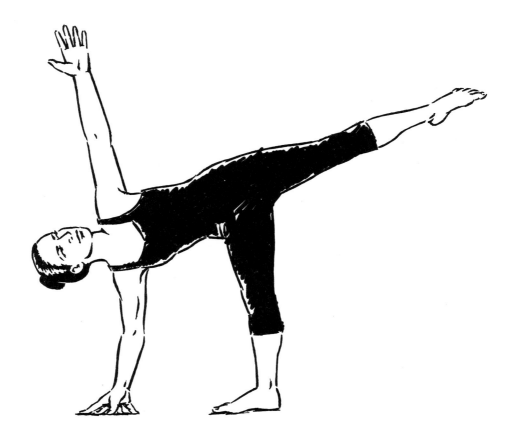

Half Moon
Ardha Candrsana

Lengthens the spine and focuses the brain on balancing

Stand on the right leg, broadening the ball of the right foot. Lengthen the left leg up behind you as you bend forwards. Inhale while lifting the right hip bone, supporting yourself with the right hand on the floor. Lengthen the left hand upwards and gently look up from the base of the skull. Inhale and exhale deeply five times, then change sides and repeat.

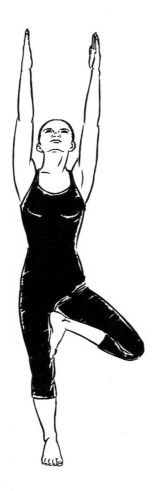

Tree Pose
Vrikshasana

Strengthens the legs and spine and gives clarity to the mind

Stand on both feet with the hands on the hips and inhale. As you exhale, lift the left foot and place the sole on the inner right thigh. Broaden the balls of both feet to stabilize the legs. Lengthen them from the buttocks down to the heels, and the front ankles up the hips. Inhale and raise the arms above the head with the shoulders relaxed. Inhale and exhale deeply 5–10 times, then change to the other leg and repeat.

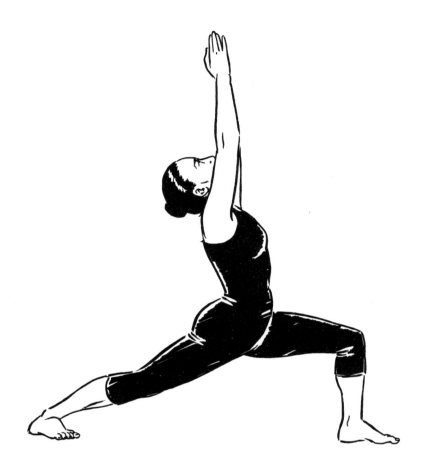

Warrior I
Virabhadrasana I

Opens the hips and strengthens the legs

From a standing position take the left leg forwards and bend the knee to 90°. Turn your right foot 75° outwards. Gently lengthen into the spine and look up from the base of the skull. Inhale and raise both hands upwards, fingers pointing skywards. Inhale and exhale deeply five times, then change sides and repeat.

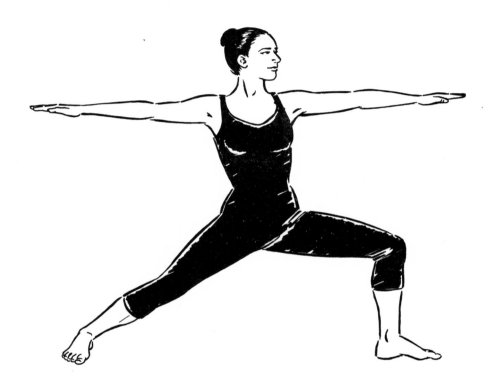

Warrior II
Virabhadrasana II

Opens the hips and strengthen the legs

From a standing position take the left leg forwards and bend the left knee to 90°. Turn the right foot behind you outwards to 75°. Lengthen the spine and look straight ahead. Inhale and raise both hands up to shoulder height. Inhale and exhale deeply five times, then change sides and repeat.

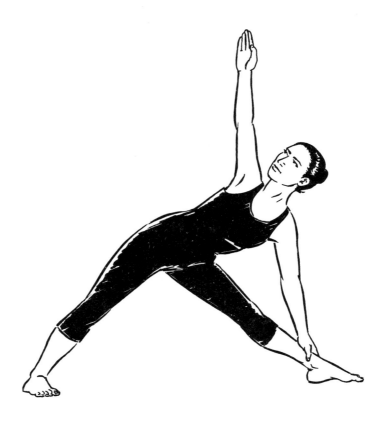

Triangle Pose
Trikonasana

Frees the pelvis and softens the lumbar spine

From a standing position take the left leg forwards. Turn the right foot behind you outwards to 75°. Inhale and engage both thighs, lengthening the legs. Exhale as you bend forwards, lifting the right hip bone up and tucking the left buttock bone underneath. Lengthen the left arm and hand along the left leg down to the outside of the ankle. Lengthen the right upwards but keep the shoulder relaxed. Looking gently upwards, inhale and exhale deeply five times. Change sides and repeat.

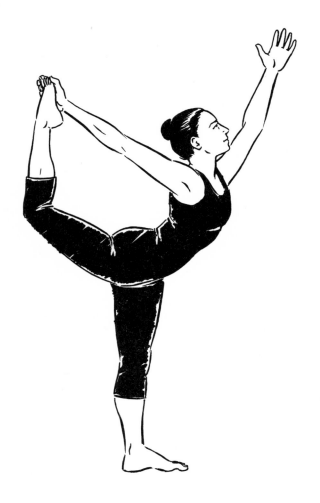

Lord of the Dance
Natarajasan

Opens the hip flexors and improves balance

Stand upright with the balls of the feet broadened. Lengthen into the legs, then inhale and lift the right leg behind you. As you exhale, grip the right ankle with the right hand. Inhale and lengthen the left arm upwards while gently looking up from the base of the skull. Inhale and exhale deeply five times. Change sides and repeat.

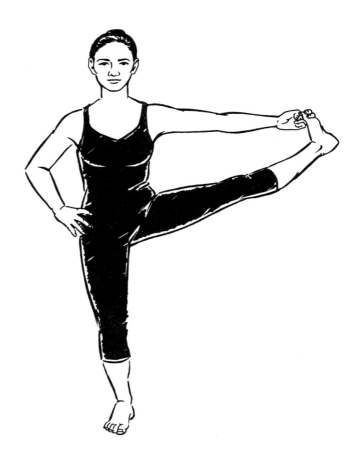

Extended Hand to Big Toe
Utthita Hasta Padangustasana

Lengthens the hamstrings and strengthens the spine

From a standing position, inhale and lift the left leg in front of you. Grip the neck of the big toe with the index finger and thumb of your left hand and exhale. Inhale, lengthen the spine, then rotate the leg towards the left, keeping the right leg straight. Inhale and exhale deeply five times. Change sides and repeat.

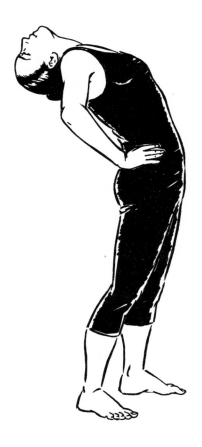

Half Wheel I
Ardhachakrasana I

Opens the front of the body stretching the abdomen and heart

Stand with both feet hip-width apart with the hands on the lower back and
the thumbs supporting the sacrum (the triangular bone at the base of the
spine and at the upper and back part of the pelvic cavity). Bend the knees
slightly as you inhale and lift the head up and then back. Exhale and lift
the trunk upwards and backwards, supporting the lower spine
by lengthening the legs. Hold the position while you inhale and exhale
deeply five times.

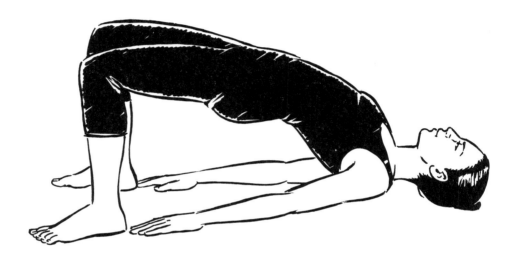

Half Wheel II
Ardhachakrasana II

Induces calm

Lie on the floor on your back with your feet hip-width apart, with both hands flat on the floor and the shoulders broad. Inhale and broaden the front of the trunk. Exhale and curl the pubic bone skywards, keeping the lower spine soft as you lift your buttocks and spine from the floor. Hold the position, inhaling and exhaling 5–15 times.

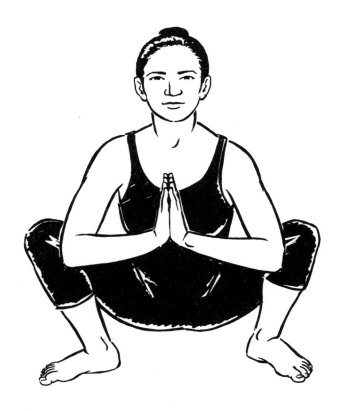

Garland
Malasana

Deeply opens the lower spine and hip flexors

Stand with the feet one-and-a-half times the width of the shoulders apart. Inhale as you bring your bottom right down and squat, keeping your heels flat on the floor. Exhale and bring the hands together in front of you into the namaste position, or as if you are praying. Keep the front ribcage open. Inhale and exhale deeply five times holding this positon.

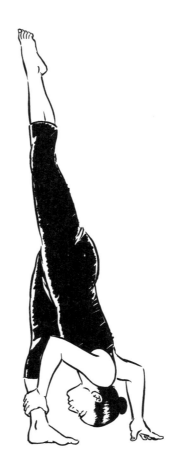

Standing Split
Urdhva Prasarita Eka

Lengthens the hamstring and opens the hips

Stand with the feet together, then bend forwards. Grasp the back of the left calf with the right hand and raise the right leg upwards to the sky. Place the left hand on the floor for support. Inhale and exhale deeply five times, then change sides and repeat.

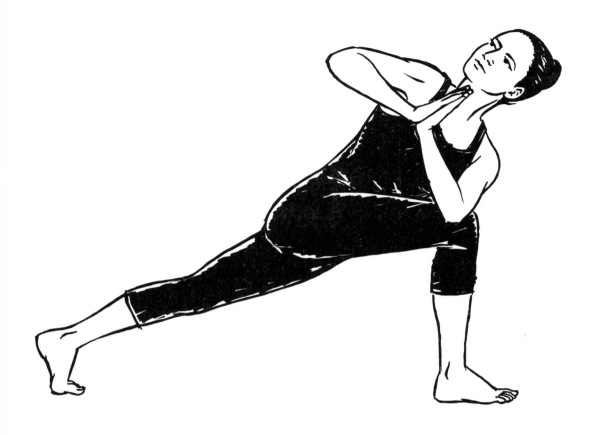

Prayer Twist
Namaskar parsvakonasana
Builds strength and releases the spine

Stand with the right leg extended forwards. Bend the knee to a
90° angle. With the left leg extended out behind you lift the left heel from
the floor. Inhale and extend both arms forwards. As you exhale, place the
left elbow on the outside of the right knee and bring the right palm down
on to the left palm while twisting the trunk round to the right and looking
gently upwards. Hold the position as you inhale and exhale five times.
Change sides and repeat.

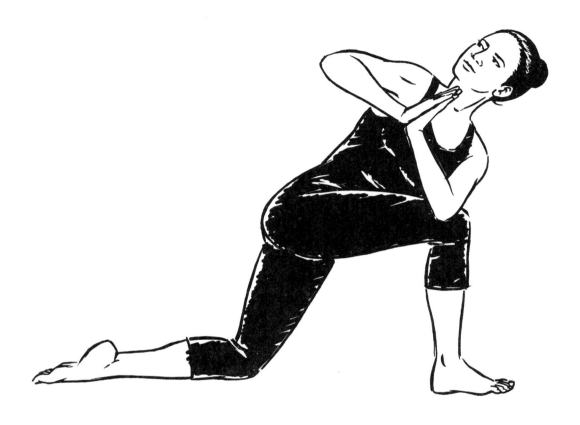

Half Prayer Twist
Ardha nam askar parsvakonasana

Increases spinal mobility and releases the hip

Stand with the right leg extended forwards. Bend the right knee to a
90° angle. Lower the left knee on to the floor, allowing the hips to open
forwards. Place the left elbow onto the right outer knee and bring the right
palm down on to the left palm while twisting the trunk round to the right
and looking gently upwards. Hold the position as you inhale and exhale
5–10 times. Change sides and repeat.

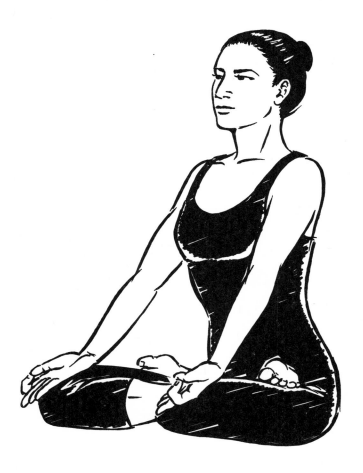

Lotus
Padmasana

Opens the pelvis and knees and softens the lumbar spine
(Not recommended for beginners or those with knee problems.)

In a sitting position inhale and lift the right leg by the shin. Fold the right
foot in towards the left hip, ensuring the ankle is supported and not
twisted, then exhale. Inhale and lift the left leg by the shin to fold the left
foot up by the right hip bone and exhale.

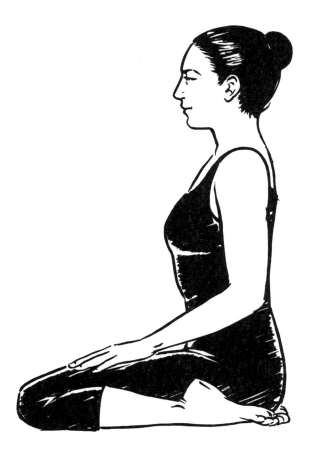

Hero's Pose
Virasana

Softens the lower back and lengthens the quadriceps

Sit with the knees bent and your bottom on the floor in between the feet, which should be slightly wider than hip-width apart. Inhale and lengthen through the spine. Exhale and lengthen the abdomen. Place the hands in a relaxed position on the thighs. Hold the position and slowly inhale and exhale deeply ten times.

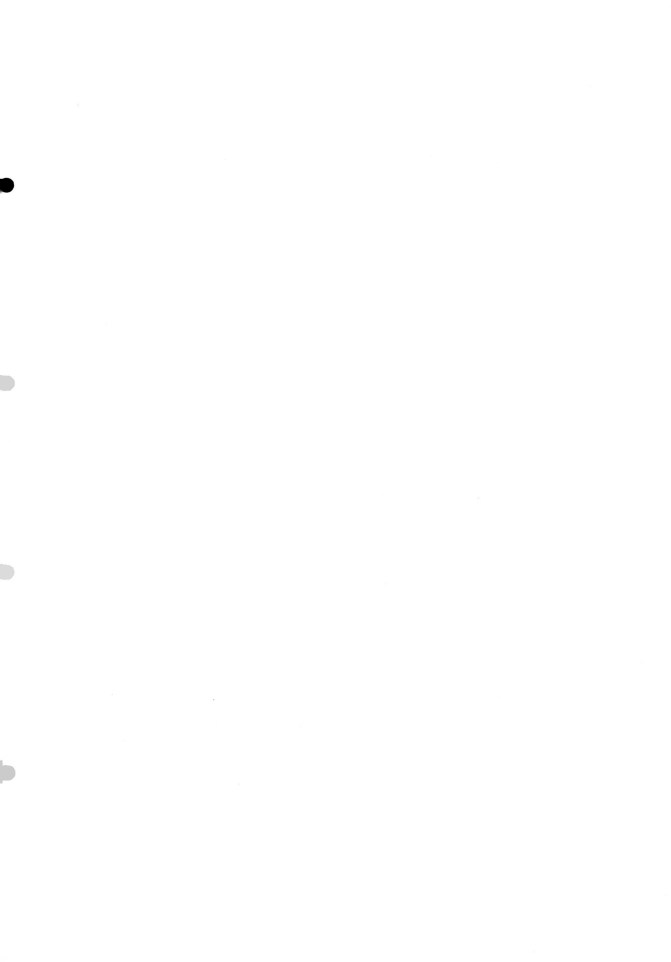

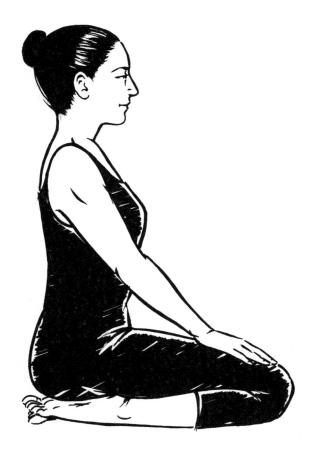

Thunderbolt
Vajrasana

Opens the hips and thighs
(Not recommended for those with knee problems.)

Kneel, then gently cross the ends of your feet behind you. Lower your bottom onto the backs of the legs, allowing the lower spine to take up its natural curve. Place the hands on the thighs, inhale and lengthen the spine. As you exhale, allow the jaw to drop slightly. Inhale and exhale deeply and slowly 5–10 times.

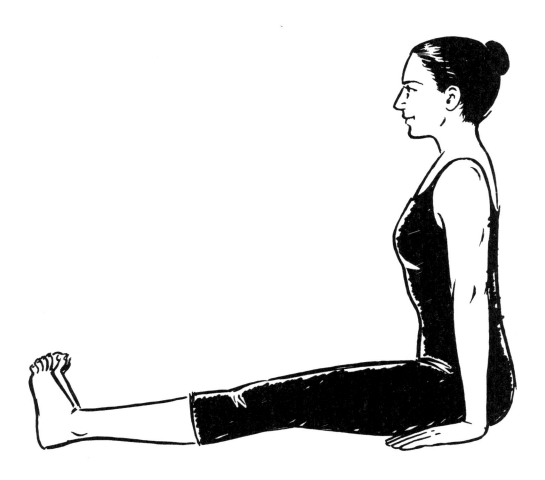

Staff
Dandasana

Releases the lower spine and lengthens the hamstrings

Sit with the legs extended in front of you. Roll the shin bones into towards each other, releasing the lower back. Lengthen from the front ankle up to the hip bones and from the buttocks down to the heels. Broaden the balls of the feet and press the hands flat and broadly into the floor by your side. Inhale up into the spine and, as you exhale, maintain a long abdomen. Hold the position, inhaling and exhaling slowly five times.

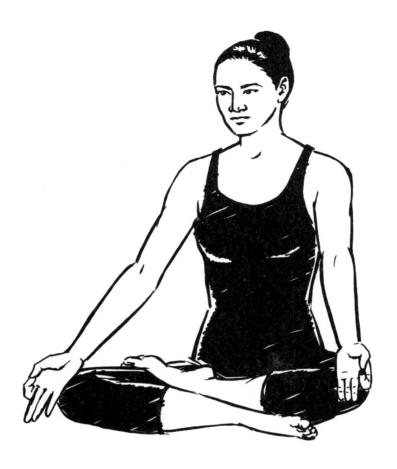

Prosperous/Auspicious
Swastikasana

Induces clarity and relaxation and stills the mind

Sit cross-legged with the left ankle resting gently on the inner right thigh.
Inhale and lengthen the spine, then exhale and maintain a long abdomen.
Lengthen through both the arms and broaden the finger bases connecting
thumb and first finger. Relax the eyes and inhale and exhale deeply
10–15 times.

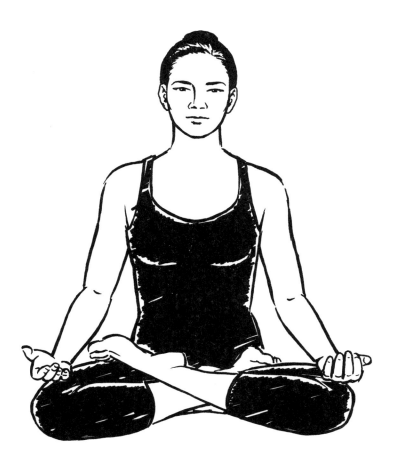

Balance
Samasana

Induces clarity and relaxation and stills the mind

Sit on the floor, gently lift the right ankle and rest it on the left inner thigh, taking care to protect the knees from twisting. (Ensure the hip is open enough to do this comfortably.) Lift the left ankle and rest it on the right inner thigh. Rest the hands, palm upwards, on the knees and inhale and lengthen into the spine. Inhale and exhale deeply 5–15 times.

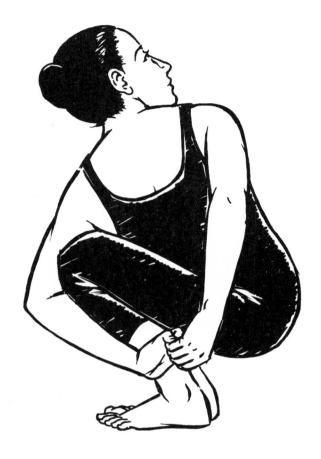

Noose
Pasasana

Increases shoulder flexibility and opens the lower back

Squat down with both heels flat on the floor and the feet close together.
Inhale and twist your trunk so that the outer left arm rests on the outer
right knee. With the right hand grip the fingers of the left hand behind you,
using a twisting motion. Inhale and exhale five times, then change sides
and repeat.

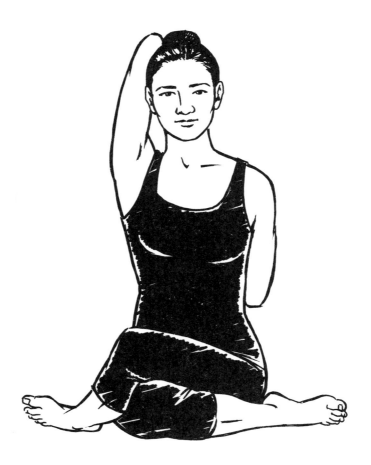

Cow Pose
Gomukhasana

Frees the pelvis deeply and opens the hip sockets

Sit with the left leg bent over the right leg with both feet broad and open. Inhale and raise both arms upwards. As you exhale, take the right arm down the middle of the back and bring the left arm underneath and grasp the palms together. Keep the right elbow pointing towards the sky, maintain a long vertical spine and relax deeply into the hips. Inhale and exhale deeply ten times, change sides and repeat.

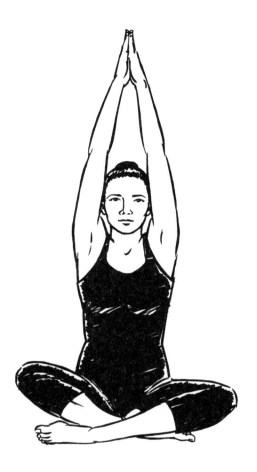

Mountain
Parvatasana

Opens the hips and lengthens the spine

Sit in a cross-legged position, inhale and extend both arms upwards, keeping the shoulders relaxed, lifting the jaw slightly and looking straight ahead. Hold the position and inhale and exhale deeply 5–10 times. You can perform this pose with the fingers intertwined or with the palms joined together, fingers stretched straight upwards.

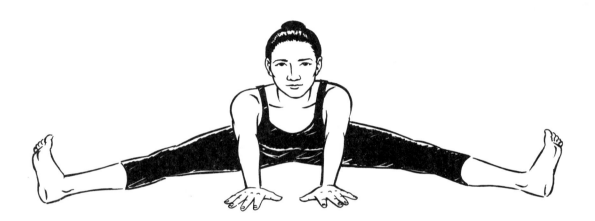

Wide-Angled Seated Forwards Bend
Upavistha Konasana

Opens the groin and lengthens the hamstrings

Sit with your legs as wide as is comfortable with the balls of the feet broad
and open. Inhale and raise the arms upwards, then exhale and lengthen
both the hands and arms forwards and then down onto the floor in front
of you. Keep the spine long and the jaw soft. Hold the position as you
inhale and exhale 5–10 times.

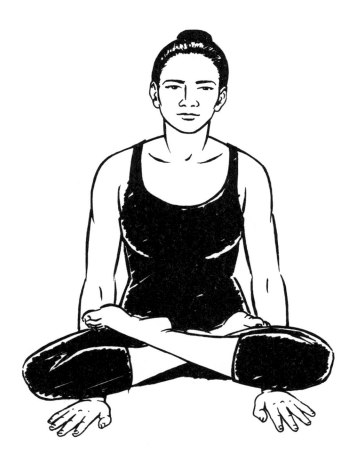

Lifted Lotus
Padmasana (Utthit)
Improves upper body strength and hip mobility

In a sitting position, lift the right ankle and rest it on the left inner thigh taking care to protect the knees from twisting. (Ensure the hip is open enough to do this comfortably.) Then lift the left ankle and rest it on the right inner thigh. Place your hands with the palms facing downwards on the floor close to you. Inhale and lengthen into the spine, lifting the body from the floor, and then exhale. Inhale and exhale five times.

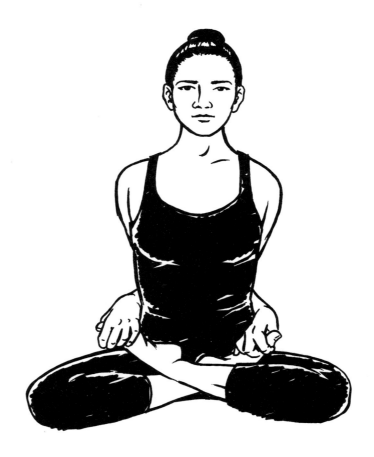

Tied Lotus
Padmasana (Baddha)

Opens the chest and shoulder and increases hip mobility

In a sitting position, lift the right ankle and rest it on the left inner thigh, taking care to protect the knees from twisting. (Ensure the hip is open enough to do this comfortably.) Then lift the left ankle and rest it on the right inner thigh. Wrap the right arm behind you, around your spine, taking hold of the left foot and wrap the left arm around the spine, taking hold of the right foot. Inhale and exhale five times in this position.

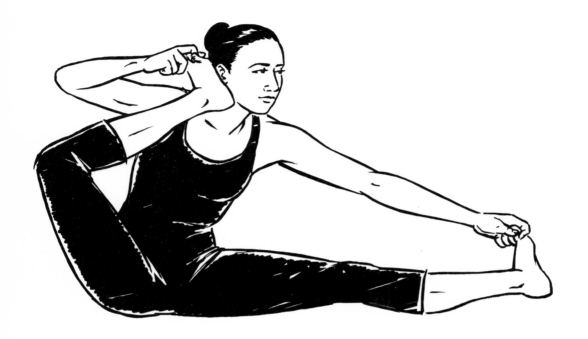

Type 1 Bow Pose in Sitting
Akarna Dhanurasana

Stretches the muscles, hip joints and shoulders, easing joint pain
and rheumatism

In a sitting position, bend forwards while exhaling. Grasp the big toe of
each foot, wrapping your middle and index finger around each toe. Your
thumb should rest on the nail root of your big toe. Inhaling, bend the knee
of the right leg and bring the foot closer to your ear by pulling on the toe.
Keep the left leg lying flat on the floor, still holding the toe with your other
hand. Hold the position and your breath. Then exhale slowly as you return
the leg to the floor. Repeat with the other leg.

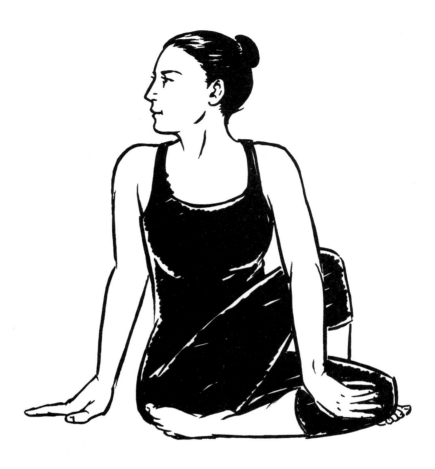

Half Spinal Twist
Ardhamatsyendrasana

Increases spinal mobility and releases the shoulders

In a sitting position, wrap the right leg over the left leg and tuck the left foot under the right buttock. Inhale and raise both arms upwards. As you exhale, place the left arm on the front of the right knee and place the left hand on the floor in line with the sacrum. Bring the jaw to the right shoulder, keeping the jaw parallel to the floor. Hold the position as you inhale and exhale 5–10 times.

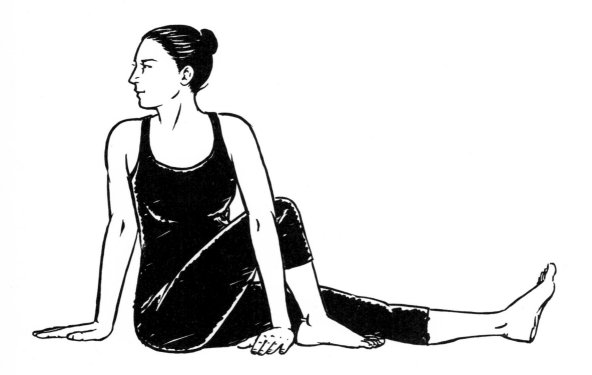

Twisted Pose I
Vakrasana

Increases mobility in the lower and upper spine and opens the hips

Sit with the legs extended out in front of you, then bend the right leg and place the right foot flat on the floor next to the left inner knee. Broaden the ball of the right foot. Inhale and raise both arms upwards. As you exhale, lower the arms, placing the right arm on the floor behind you in line with the sacrum and the left hand alongside the outside of the right knee with the palm flat on the floor. Hold the position as you inhale and exhale 5–10 times, then change sides and repeat.

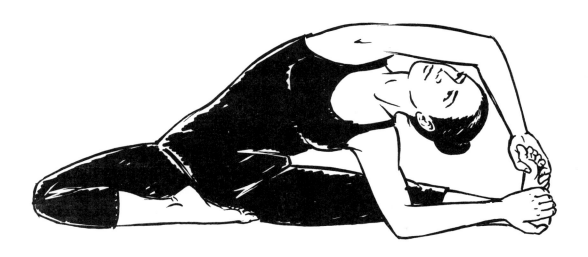

Revolved Head to Knee
Parivrtta Janu Sirsasana

Increases spinal mobility and opens the waist and abdomen

Sit with the legs wide open, then bend the right leg to bring the right foot towards the groin. Keep the left leg extended out wide. Inhale and raise both arms upwards. As you exhale, lengthen the spine over towards the left and grip the left foot. Hold the position as you inhale and exhale 5–10 times, then change sides and repeat.

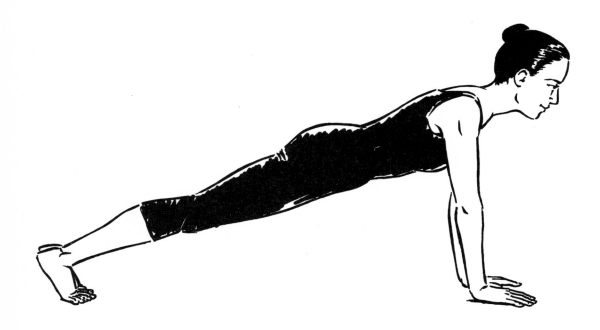

Plank
Adho Vitiyasana
Strength and spine stability

From an all-fours position, extend the legs out behind you and lengthen from the front ankles up to the hip bones and from the buttocks down to the heels. With the hands under shoulders, broaden the finger bases and keep neck loose. Hold the position as you inhale and exhale 5–10 times and then rest.

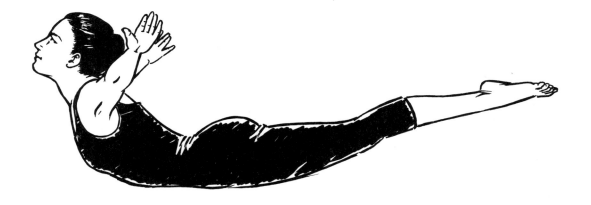

Locust
Salambhasana

Enhances mood, self-esteem and general confidence, opens the heart centre and aids digestion

Lie flat on your front and inhale. As you exhale, lengthen through the front of your body from the pubic bone to the throat and lengthen the legs out of the pelvis. Extend your arms out to the sides and back slightly as if flying and lift your head, upper torso, arms and legs away from the floor. Use the core muslces to support the spinal column from collapsing. Look up gently and hold the position as you inhale and exhale 5–10 times, then slowly release downwards.

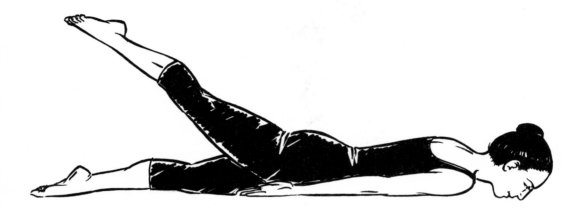

Half Locust
Shalabhasana Half

Core strength, and spinal stability

Lie flat on your front and inhale. As you exhale, engage the abdomen and
lengthen from the front of the right ankle up to your hip bones, keeping
the trunk broad and open with your face down and neck loose. Keep the
palms broad underneath the pelvis. Hold the position as you inhale and
exhale 5–10 times and then repeat with the other side.

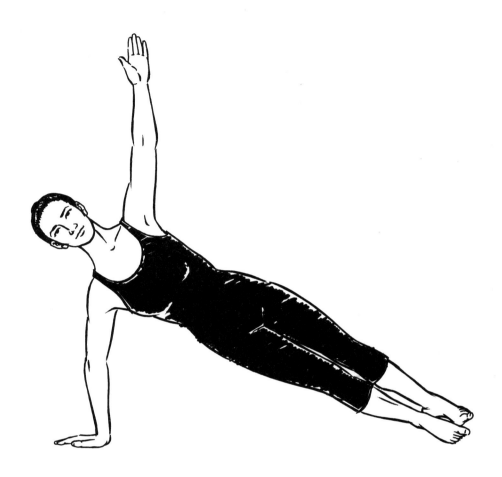

Side Plank
Vasisthasana

Strengthens the side waist, enhancing lateral balance and muscle tone

Lie on your right side. Place the right hand underneath the right shoulder and stack the legs one on top of the other. Use the core muscles to lift the hips off the floor, keeping the head in line with the rest of the body. Hold the position as you inhale and exhale 5–10 times.

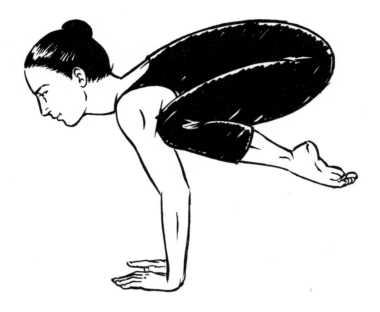

Crane/Birdie
Bakasana

Strengthens the upper body and improves balance

Kneel and place the hands flat on the floor in front of you with the palms
wide open and flat. Inhale and place your knees into your armpits. As you
exhale, use the abdominal muscles to lift the weight of the body upwards
off the floor, supported by the hands. Breathe and maintain the lift and
look gently forwards. Hold the position as you inhale and exhale
5–10 times.

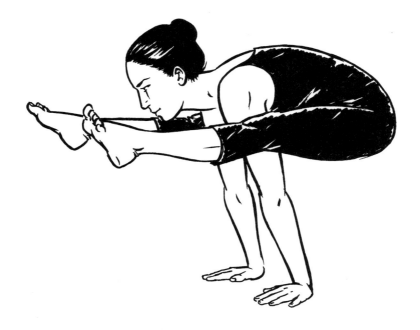

Firefly
Tittibhasana

Benefits shoulder and upper body strength and tones the core muscles

In a sitting position with the legs open and the arms directly underneath the shoulders, place the hands flat on the floor between the legs. Inhale and, as you exhale, stack one leg at a time over the upper arms. Press the arms against the legs at the same time as pressing the legs into the arms and slightly looking forwards. Broaden the feet to activate the legs. Hold the position as you inhale and exhale 5–10 times.

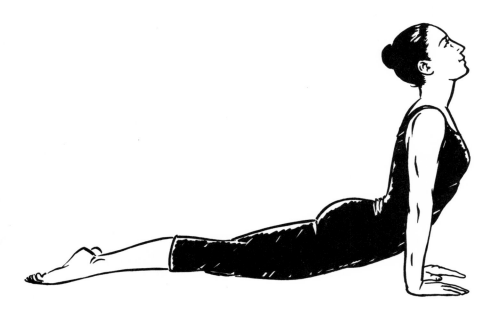

Upwards-Facing Dog
Urdvha Mukha Svanasana

Lengthens abdomen and upper body, releases the shoulders
and aids digestion (Not recommended for those with back pain)

Lie flat on the front of the body. Place the hands, palms flat, by the sides
of the ribcage so there is a vertical line between the elbow and the hand
and inhale. As you exhale, separate the ribs from the abdomen using the
breathing and lift the trunk off the floor. Draw the shoulders away from the
ears and support your weight on the arms. Hold the position, then inhale
and exhale five times only.

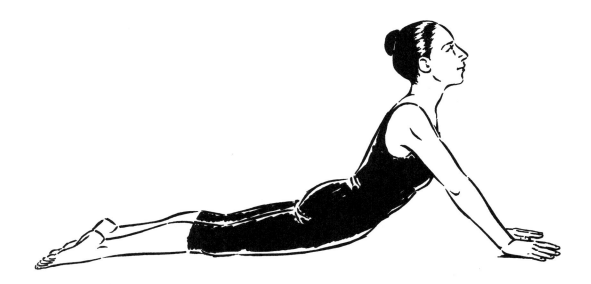

Cobra
Bhujangasana

Aids digestion, lengthens the abdomen and increases spine mobility

Lie flat on the front of the body with the hands extended forwards as far away from body as possible while. Inhale and, as you exhale, lift the upper ribs away from the abdomen and lift the trunk up from the floor. Lengthen from the front ankles up to the hip bones. Hold the position as you inhale and exhale 5–10 times.

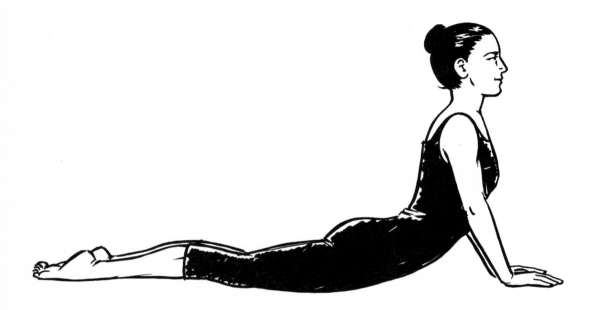

Cobra Variation II
Dwipadsahajhasta Bhujangasana
Increases spine mobility and aids digestion

Lie flat on the front of the body with the hands extended slightly out in front of the shoulders and inhale. As you exhale, lift the upper ribs away from the abdomen and the trunk away from the floor. Lengthen from the front ankles up to the hip bones. Hold the position as you inhale and exhale 5–10 times.

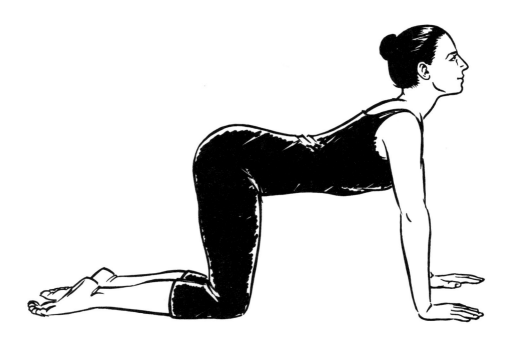

Cow
Bitilasana

Increases spine integrity and core strength

In an all-fours position, place the hands underneath the shoulders, and the knees underneath the hip bones. Inhale and broaden the finger bases. Exhale and engage the abdomen. Inhale and lift the head from the base of the skull, exhale and lengthen into the spine. Hold the position as you inhale and exhale 5–10 times.

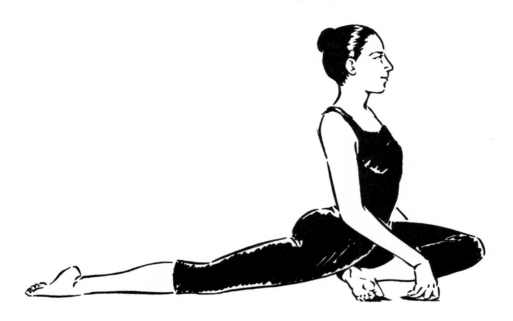

Pigeon
Eka Pada Rajakapotasana

Increases hip flexor flexibility and frees the spine

From a sitting position, bring your left knee in between your hands and extend your right leg out behind you. Inhale and lengthen the spine, and as you exhale, shift the right buttock bone backwards to open the lumbar spine. Hold the position as you inhale and exhale 5–10 times. Change sides and repeat.

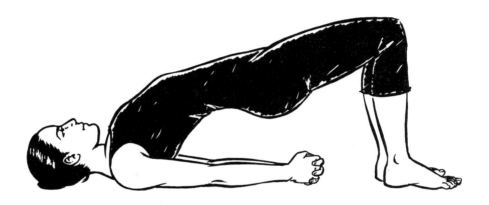

Bridge
Setu Bandha Sarvangasana

Increases spinal mobility and opens the heart and solar plexus centres

Lie on your back with the feet in line with the buttock bones. Clasp the hands together underneath your back and broaden into the backs of the shoulders. Inhale and curl the pubic bone to the sky, keeping the buttocks soft, and lift your back off the floor. Hold the position as you inhale and exhale 5–15 times, then slowly roll down.

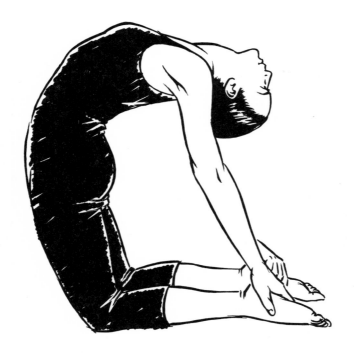

Camel
Ustrasana

Opens the yin energy channels on the front of the body
and releases shoulders and lower spine

Start from an all-fours position. Inhale and raise yourself up to a kneeling
position. Reach behind you and place the left hand on the left heel and the
right hand on the right heel, opening the heart centre. As you exhale, let
your head relax back, opening the throat centre. Hold the position as you
inhale and exhale 5–10 times and relax.

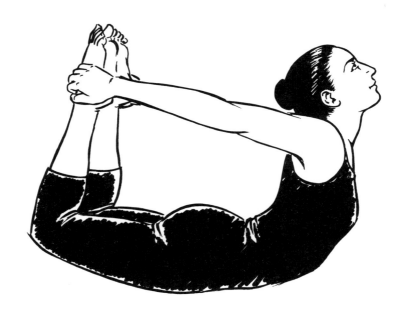

Bow
Dhanurasana

Increases spinal mobility and induces sense of well-being

Lie flat on the front of the body and inhale. As you exhale, reach behind you and grasp your ankles. Inhale and then as you exhale lift the trunk and knees away from each other, lengthening the spinal column. Hold the position as you inhale and exhale 5–10 times and then release slowly.

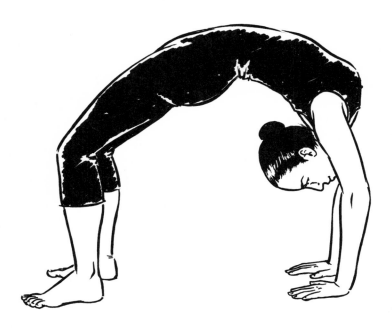

Upward Bow/Wheel
Urdhva Dhanurasana

Increases spinal flexibility and opens heart centre

Lie flat on your back and place your palms by your shoulders with your
fingers pointing towards your shoulders. Place the feet hip-width apart and
flat on the floor. Inhale and then, as you exhale, press through the hands
to lift the trunk and pelvis up to the sky. Use both feet to lift yourself. Hold
the position as you inhale and exhale 3–5 times.

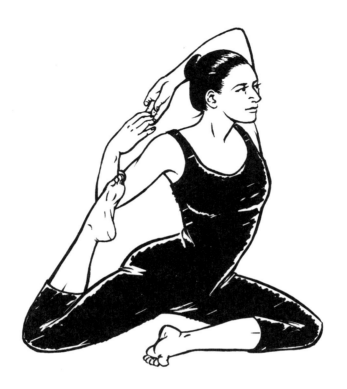

Kneeling Dancer Pose
Natarajasana

Opens the hips and shoulders, maintains pelvic mobility and spinal flexibility

Kneel with the left knee extended further in front. Inhale and raise the left arm upwards and grasp the right hand behind your back. Bend the right knee to lift the right foot and set the right elbow near the inside of the right ankle, which is drawn in towards the spine. Inhale and, as you exhale, draw the right ankle into towards the right buttock, increasing the hip stretch. Hold the position as you inhale and exhale 5–10 times.

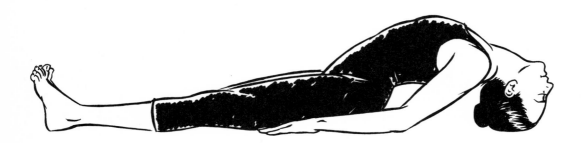

Fish

Matsyasana

Opens the throat centre and releases the lower spine

Lie flat on the floor on your back with your hands underneath your buttocks, palms down and elbows tucked in towards the sides of the body. Inhale and, as you exhale, lift the solar plexus towards the sky. Keep breathing into your elongated trunk and relax the head back to rest the crown on the floor. Hold the position as you inhale and exhale 5–10 times and then rest.

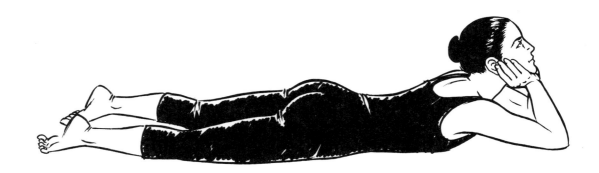

Crocodile
Makarasana

Stretches the neck and elongates the throat centre, improving circulation

Lie flat on the front of the body with the hands underneath either side of
the chin. Inhale and open the front chest. Then, as you exhale, lift the head
and look upwards. Hold the position as you inhale and exhale
5–10 times and then rest.

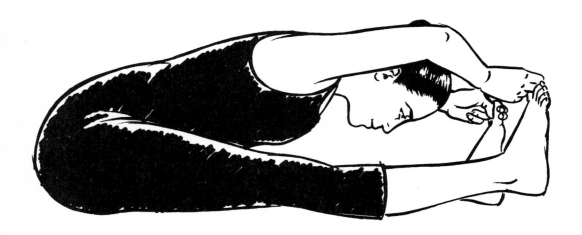

Big Toe Pose
Padangusthasana

Lengthens hamstrings and releases the lower spine

Sit with the legs extended out long in front of you. Inhale and raise both
arms upwards. As you exhale, reach down and place the index finger and
thumb of each hand around each big toe. Inhale and lengthen the spine.
As you exhale, hinge the hips forwards, keeping the back long. Hold the
position as you inhale and exhale 5–15 times.

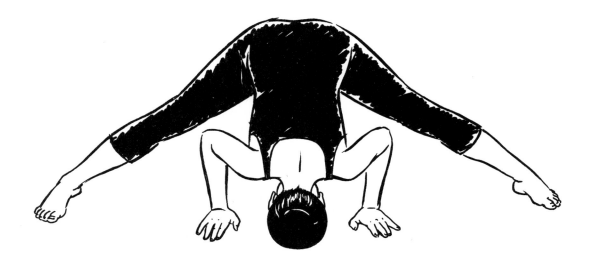

Wide-Legged Forwards Bend
Prasarita Padottanasana

Opens the groin to release the pelvis and hips

Stand upright with the feet parallel and as wide apart as comfortably possible and inhale. As you exhale, reach down and place the hands flat on the floor in front of you, bending the knees if required. Inhale to open the front of the trunk and, as you exhale, bend further to open the spine. Hold the position as you inhale and exhale 5–15 times.

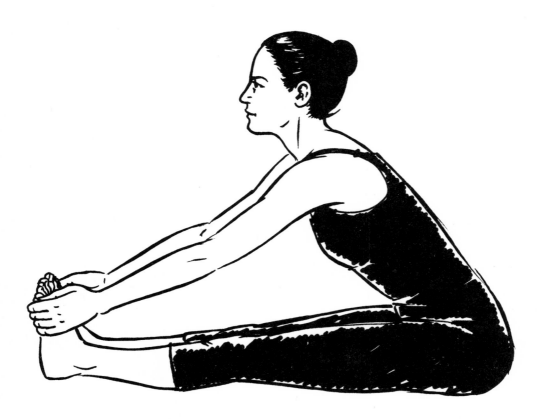

Seated Forwards Bend
Sharanagata Mudra

Lengthens the hamstrings and opens the lower spine

Sit with the legs extended out long in front of you. Roll the shin bones
towards each other to release the sacrum. Inhale, bend forwards and
place the hands around the outside of the feet, keeping the spine
long on the exhalation. Hold the position as you inhale and exhale
5–15 times.

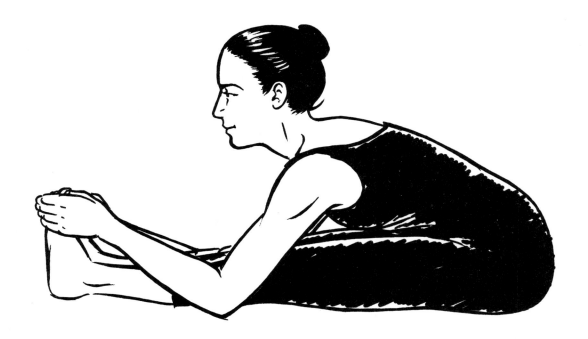

Seated Forwards Bend
Paschimottanasana (Full)

Lengthens the hamstrings and opens the lower spine

Sit with the legs extended out long in front of you. Roll the shin bones towards each other to release the sacrum. Inhale, bend forwards and place the hands around the outside of the feet, keeping the spine long on the exhalation. Inhale and draw the ribs towards the thighs. Hold the position as you inhale and exhale 5–15 times.

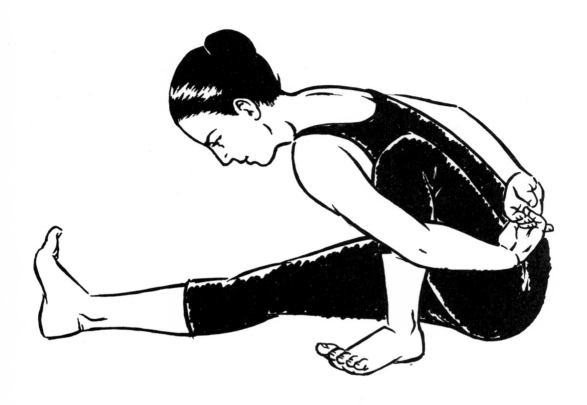

Marichi I
Marichyasana I

Releases the spine and opens the shoulder

From a sitting position, bend the right knee to bring the right foot into the right buttock, broadening the balls of the feet. Inhale and raise both arms upwards. Then, as you exhale, wrap the right arm around the spine and grip the left hand. Inhale and lengthen the trunk forwards. Hold the position as you inhale and exhale 5–10 times, then change sides.

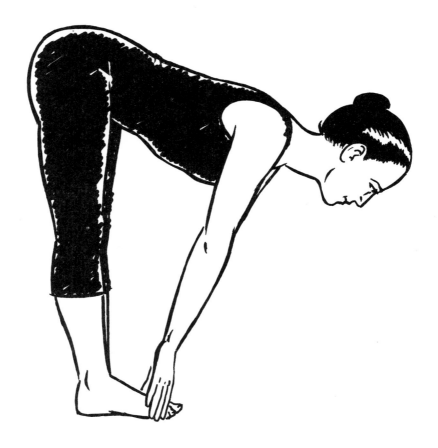

Standing Half-Forwards Bend
Ardha Uttanasana

Lengthens hamstrings

Stand with the feet together or hip-width apart. Inhale and, as you exhale, bend forward, keeping the knees slightly soft. Inhale as you extend the trunk away from the legs. Exhale and lift the buttocks up away from the ground. Hold the position as you inhale and exhale five times.

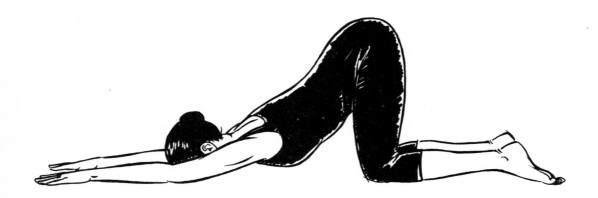

Extended Puppy
Uttana Shishosana

Releases the spine and opens the chest

Kneel on all fours and then extend the arms forwards with the hands flat on the ground. Inhale and, as you exhale, lift the sacrum skywards as you open the chest to the Earth. Hold the position as you inhale and exhale 5–15 times.

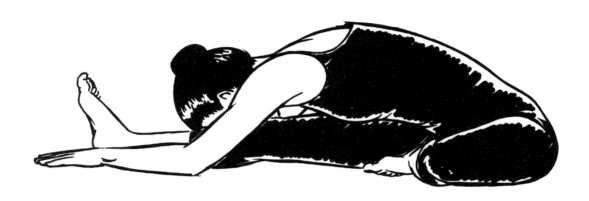

Head-to-Knee Forwards Bend
Janu Sirsasana

Elongates the hamstring and opens the lower spine

Sit with the right leg extended out in front of you and the left foot tucked into the right inner thigh. Lengthen both legs in both positions. Inhale and raise the arms upwards. As you exhale, lengthen the trunk over the right leg, keeping the ribcage open and place both hands flat on the floor on either side of the right leg. Hold the position as you inhale and exhale 5–15 times.

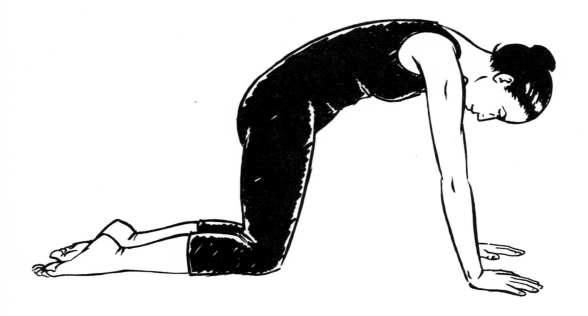

Cat
Marjaryasana
Increases spinal mobility

Kneel in an all-fours position with the hands directly under the shoulders and the knees under the hip bones. Inhale and, as you exhale, roll the spine up towards the sky. Let the head relax and drop as you release the spine. Hold the position as you inhale and exhale 5–10 times.

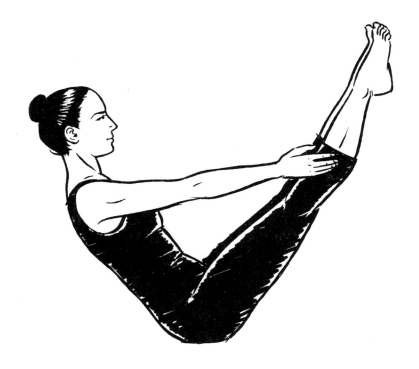

Full Boat
Paripurna Navasana
Strengthens the abdomen and spine

Sit on the sitting bones, inhale and extend both legs upwards. Reach up and touch the outside of the calves with the fingers. Keep the jaw parallel to the gound. As you exhale, engage the abdomen by keeping the spine long. Hold the legs firmly together as you inhale and exhale 5–15 times.

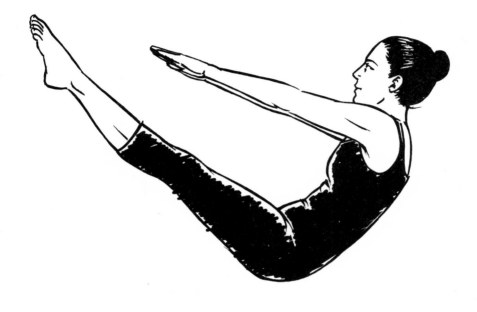

Boat

Noukasana

Strengthens the abdomen and spine

Sit on the sitting bones, inhale and extend both legs upwards. Keep the jaw parallel to the ground. As you exhale engage the abdomen by keeping the spine long. Relax into the spine a little by drawing the ribs into the spine. Keep the legs firmly together, look up gently and hold the position as you inhale and exhale 5–15 times.

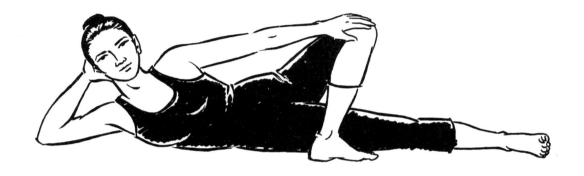

Side-Reclining Leg Lift
Anantasana I

Lengthens the inner thighs and opens the waist muscles

Lie out straight on the right-hand side with the head propped up on the elbow. Lengthen the right leg and bend the left leg over the right. Place the left foot flat on the floor in front of the right knee with the toes facing towards the right foot and the knee pointing to the sky. Rest the left hand on the left knee to keep the hip joint open. Hold the position as you inhale and exhale 5–10 times and then change sides.

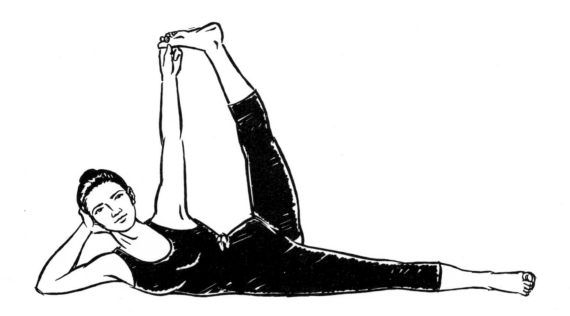

Side-Reclining Leg Lift II
Anantasana II

Opens the inner thighs and hamstrings

Lie straight out on the right-hand side. Hold the weight of the head in the right hand by resting on the right elbow, placing the right hand just behind the ear with the fingers spread open. Lift the left leg straight upwards and grip the neck of the big toe with the thumb and index finger of the left hand. Extend the left leg while keeping the right leg lengthened. Hold the position as you inhale and exhale 5–10 times. Change sides and repeat.

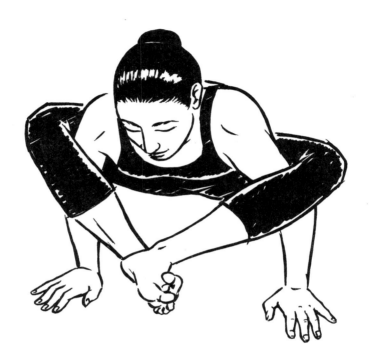

Shoulder-Pressing Pose
Bhujapidasana

Strenthens upper body and arms

Starting from a squatting position with the hands flat on the floor, inhale as you wrap the right leg around the outside of the right arm and the left leg around the outside of the left arm. Exhale as you lift the body from the floor. Hold the position as you inhale and exhale five times only.

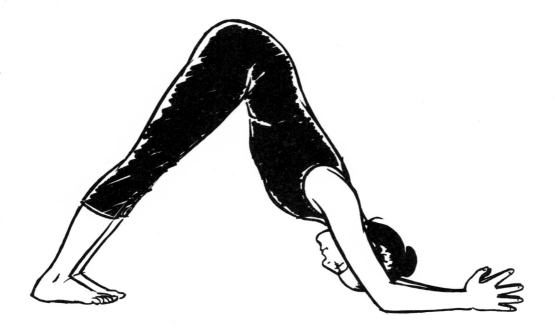

Dolphin
Makarasana

Lengthens the spine and hamstrings

From an all-fours position on the elbows inhale and, as you exhale, lift the tailbone to the sky, lengthening the spine and waist muscles. Lift the buttocks upwards, keep the heels flat on the floor and lift from the front ankle up to the hip bones. Keep the hands alive and bases of the fingers open. Hold the position as you inhale and exhale 5–15 times.

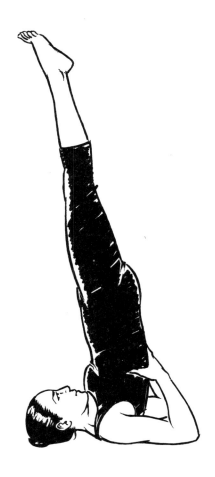

Shoulder Stand
Sarvangasana

Calms the nervous system and increases blood flow to the brain

Lie flat on your on your back and inhale. As you exhale, lift the legs up to the sky and support them by broadening into the shoulder blades. Place the hands on the lower back and allow your breathing to be free and easy. Keep lengthening through the spine to lengthen the legs upwards. Hold the position as you inhale and exhale 15–30 times.

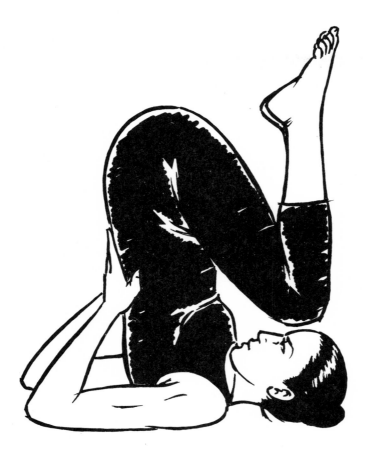

Horse Gesture in Shoulder Stand
Ashwini Mudra

Increases blood supply to the liver and releases the lower spine

Lie flat on your back, inhale and bring the knees to the forehead,
supporting the spine with both hands. Keeping the buttocks close to the
heels, exhale and then enjoy deep breaths while lifting the spine upwards,
broadening the backs of the shoulders to support the weight. Hold the
position as you inhale and exhale 5–30 times.

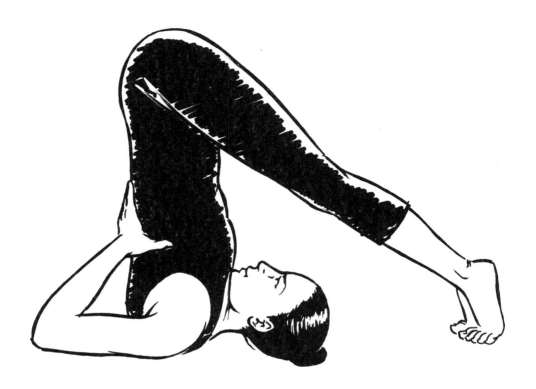

Plough
Arda Halasana

Releases the lower spine, lengthens and relaxes the spinal column, calms the nervous system and relaxes the facial muscles

Lie flat on your back with the palms of the hands flat on the floor and inhale. As you exhale, bring the knees to the chest and inhale again. Exhale and bring your knees to your forehead. Place your hands flat on your lower spine and inhale. As you exhale, take the feet over the head to touch the floor behind you. If your feet do not touch the floor, do not force them. Relax and inhale into the ribcage. As you exhale, engage the abdomen so that the spine lengthens. Relax here as you inhale and exhale 15–20 times, then roll down slowly.

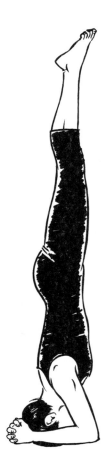

Supported Headstand
Salamba Sirsasana

Increases blood flow to the brain and face

From an all-fours position, place the elbows on the floor directly under
the shoulders. Place the crown of the head on the floor and interlock the
fingers around the skull to support it. Inhale and, as you exhale, gently
engage the abdomen to lift the legs slowly together to an upright position.
Hold the position as you inhale and exhale 5–30 times.

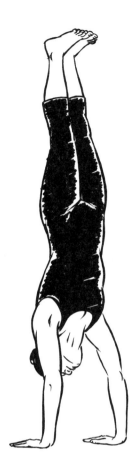

Downwards-Facing Tree Handstand
Adho Mukha Vrksasan

Strengthens the arms and abdomen and increases blood flow to the brain

Stand upright and then bend forwards to place both hands flat on the floor, broadening the bases of the fingers. Inhale and, as you exhale, gently lift one leg and then the other into an upright position. Hold the legs together firmly as you inhale and exhale five times.

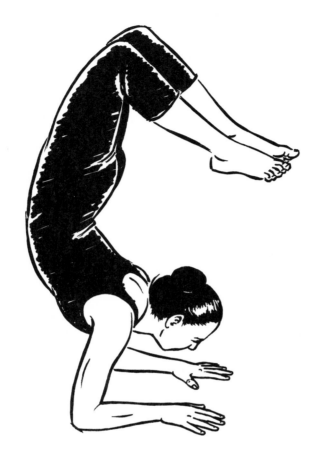

Scorpion
Vrischikasana

Opens the chest and shoulders

Starting from an all-fours position, lower the elbows to the floor directly below the shoulders, place the palms out flat and broaden the bases of the fingers. Inhale and, as you exhale, gently lift both legs in an upright position, bending the knees so the flats of the feet are directly over the head. Hold the position as you inhale and exhale 5–10 times.

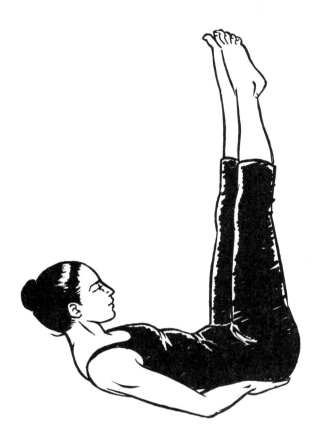

Leg-Raise (with both legs and one leg)
Uttanpadasana

Improves abdominal strength

Lie flat on your back with the hands placed palms-down under the lower
spine for support. Gently lift the legs upwards and inhale. Exhale as you
lift the trunk slowly off of the floor. Keep the jaw parallel with the floor as
you look straight ahead. Hold the position, inhale and exhale freely
10 times, release and lower the truck and legs back to the floor.

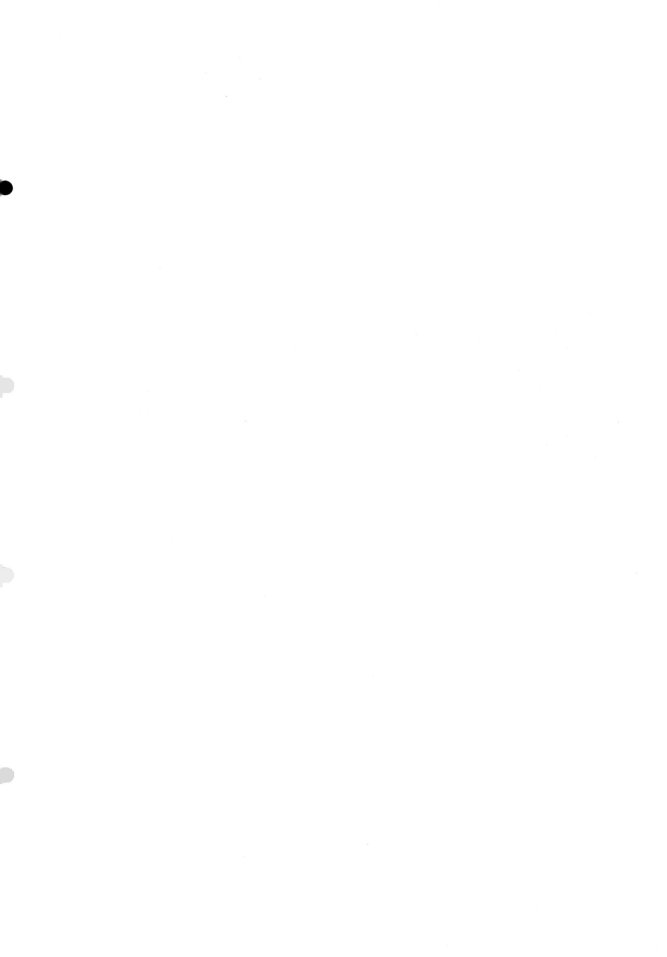

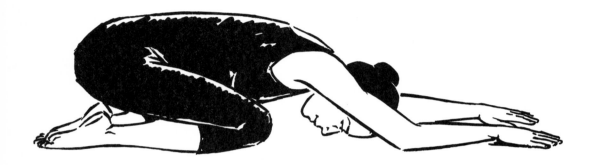

Child's Pose
Balasana

Helps relieve stress, mild depression, headache, fatigue and insomnia

Kneel on the floor with the feet together but the thighs hip-width apart. Lower your bottom until it touches the heels. Exhale as you bend at the back of the waist and allow your hips to sink down toward the floor. As you inhale, notice your stomach expand against your thighs. Either stretch the arms in front of you with the palms toward the floor or bring the arms back alongside the thighs with the palms facing upwards. Do whichever is more comfortable to you. Inhale and lengthen your neck, placing your forehead on the floor (or a mat or cushion). Exhale and allow the weight of your shoulders to fall freely towards the floor.

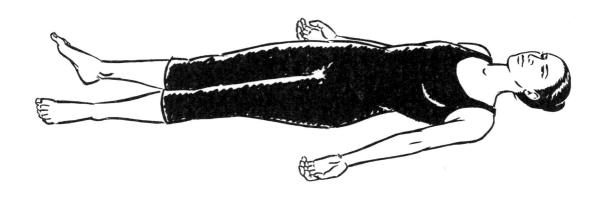

Corpse
Savasana

Stimulates blood circulation, improves concentration and relieves fatigue, nervousness, asthma, constipation, diabetes, indigestion, and insomnia

Lie flat on your back and let your feet to roll out to either side. Bring your arms alongside, but slightly separated from, your body, palms facing upwards, fingers slightly curled and relaxed. Relax your whole body, including your face. Let your body feel heavy. Breathe naturally.

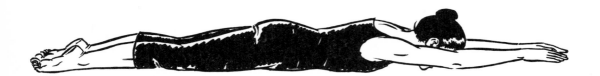

Reversed Corpse
Adhvasana

Induces relaxation

Lie flat on your front and relax deeply into the small curve of your lower spine, placing the arms and legs wherever you are most comfortable. Imagine yourself dropping deeply into the Earth, relaxing every muscle and bone. Hold the position for 10–20 minutes.

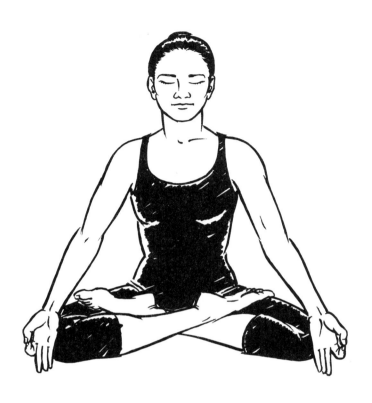

Meditation
Dhyan Mudra

Stills the mind and aids concentration

Sit with the right foot on the left inner thigh and the left foot on the right inner thigh ensuring that the legs are turned from the hips. Rest the backs of hands, palms facing outwards and broadened, on the ends of the knees with the index finger softly touching the thumb. Lengthen from the armpits to the hip bones. Keep the jaw parallel to the ground. Hold for 10–30 minutes, focusing on relaxed and easy breathing.

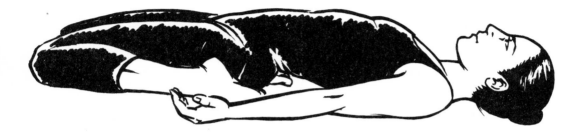

Reclining Hero
Supta Virasana

Opens the quadriceps and the front heart

Lie flat on your back, then bend the knees and tuck the feet up under the
buttocks. Gently roll the spine to the floor, releasing and dropping into
the lower spine. Allow the knees to be heavy, but if there is any pain in the
knees do not continue this posture. Hold for as long as it is comfortable.

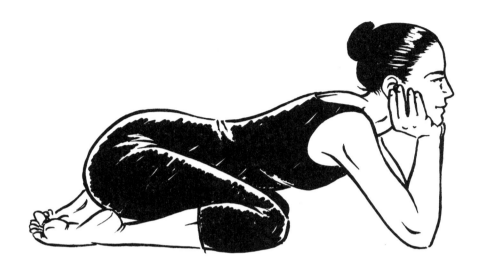

Propped Rabbit
Hastashirasana

Opens the lower back and groin

Starting from an all-fours position, prop the elbows on the floor and lower the bottom onto the heels and look straight ahead. Press the chest down so that the sacrum lengthens away from the base of the skull and lengthens the spine. Hold for five breaths.

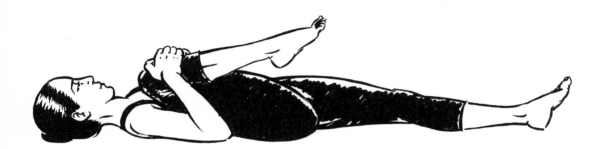

Air Release
Pavanamuktasana 1 Leg

Releases air from the body and opens the lower back

Lie flat on your back and draw the right knee up towards the chest, grasping the shin with the hands. Lengthen the left leg by stretching out the hips and press the lower spine into the floor. Keep the head relaxed and long. Hold the position and inhale and exhale 5–15 times.

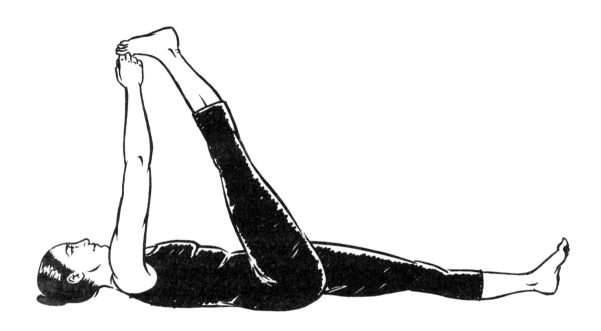

Reclining Big Toe
Supta Padangusthasana

Elongates the hamstrings and spinal column

Lie flat on your back and stretch the right leg upwards. Grip the big toe around the neck with the thumb and index finger of the right hand. Keep pressing the back of the left knee into the floor to open the lower spine. Keep the neck long and the head relaxed. Hold the position as you inhale and exhale 15 times, then change sides and repeat.

Types of Yoga

Yoga is suitable for everyone, regardless of age or ability. There are many different types of yoga, so it will be easy to find one that suits you.

Ashtanga Yoga
Ashtanga yoga, sometimes called 'power yoga', is light on meditation but heavy on developing strength and stamina. The poses are more difficult than those of other styles, and students must move quickly from one pose to the next to build strength and flexibility. Even before an Ashtanga session begins, students are taken through a warm-up to activate the muscles. The style is suitable for anyone in reasonable physical condition but should be avoided by those who are new to exercise – even the so-called 'beginner' routines offer a physically demanding workout.

Bikram Yoga
This style is also known as 'hot yoga' because it is practised in a room heated to 38°C (100°F) or higher in order to replicate the temperature of the birthplace in India of Bikram Choudhury (born 1946), the originator of this style of yoga. Bikram yoga focuses on 26 postures performed in a certain order. The exercises are very physical and the intensity is high. Combined with the heat, it makes for a tough workout. This style is recommended for yoga veterans and extremely fit individuals.

Hatha Yoga
The foundation of all other yoga styles, this mellow form of yoga concentrates on simple poses that flow from one to the next at a very comfortable pace. Participants are encouraged to move at their own speed and to take the time to focus on their breathing and meditation. The ideal way to practice Hatha yoga is to approach the session in a calm, meditative mood, which means it is ideal for winding down at the end of a tough day.

Iyengar Yoga
B.K.S. Iyengar (born 1918) founded this classical style of yoga. It is less physically demanding and so is perfect for beginners and those who haven't exercised in a while. Props such as chairs, straps, blocks and pillows, and even sandbags, are used to compensate for any lack of flexibility, which is helpful for anyone with back or joint problems. Iyengar is one of the most popular types of yoga taught today.

Jivamukti Yoga
A physically intense style of yoga, this was founded in New York City in 1984. 'Jivamukti' means liberation while living, and this style of yoga can involve music, chanting and scripture reading.

Kundalini Yoga
Known also as the 'yoga of awareness', 'Kundalini' refers to the energy of the Root chakra, which surrounds the base of the spine. The principle behind this style of yoga is the belief that freeing up this area can unleash the unlimited potential that lies within that energy centre. Kundalini yoga involves lots of core work on the abdominal muscles and around the spine and perhaps more sitting than other styles of yoga. It can be enjoyed by anyone of any age or physical ability.

Prenatal Yoga
This style of yoga is designed for expectant mothers and those who have recently given birth and want to get back into shape. It keeps the core strong, helps the posture and involves lots of breath work. Prenatal yoga offers a slower-paced workout.

Restorative Yoga
Restorative yoga is the yoga of deep, aware relaxation. It is considered the yoga of being, rather than the yoga of doing. Restorative yoga uses a sequence of three or four specially designed postures in which the body is completely supported.

There are five underlying principles to practising yoga with integrity and you will need to follow these when using this book, and also when off the yoga mat in your everyday life. Then you will invite a deep sense of connectedness to the total energy of the universe and become connected and charged to that mass of energy without compromising yourself. The yamas can be thought of as the ethical restraints that are necessary for achieving harmony with other beings.

THE FIVE UNDERLYING YAMA PRINCIPLES OF THE YOGA METHOD

● SENSITIVITY TO ALL ACTIONS AND IMPACTS (AHIMSA)

The foundation of yoga practice and teaching, ahimsa is focused through feeling the quality of awareness itself onto the actual sensations arising in the body as the direct and indirect impacts of actions being taken. Direct impacts are those sensations arising from the intended muscular events themselves. Indirect impacts are those sensations and states arising from the response to these events in connective tissue, bone, vital organs, feelings states, energy, attention, thought and awareness. It generates a clear awareness of what is actually happening.

● HONESTY ABOUT WHAT IS ACTUALLY HAPPENING (SATYA)

Satya is honoured by acknowledging that what is happening is actually happening. It is expressed through an ongoing responsiveness to internal and external events. Viewed from this perspective, it means that if an action that needs to be taken can be taken, it is taken – nothing that can be done is left undone. Likewise if an action that needs to be taken cannot be effectively taken, it cannot be taken, but the consequences of this be honoured.

● OPENNESS ABOUT WHAT IS ACTUALLY HAPPENING (ASTEYA)

Asteya is honoured by practising without any agenda except to be present to what is actually happening and what is possible (satya). This means letting go of any specific, limited intention and concentrating on what is actually happening, moment by moment. This openness is expressed through an ongoing trust in what is actually happening, culminating in the realization of the imperfectable nature of all phenomena. This displaces the grasping mind and allows space for honesty and sensitivity to function, and invites a deep trust in the indivisible unity of life functioning through the inherent integrity of the body and the inherent unity of body, mind and spirit.

● GENEROSITY TOWARDS WHAT IS ACTUALLY HAPPENING (APARIGRAHA)

Aparigraha is honoured by allowing what is actually happening to happen just as it does without any judgement. This means letting go of any evaluation of experience or action, without even judging their having arisen. It is expressed by an ongoing disidentification with experiences, perceptions and actions, culminating in the realization of the impersonal nature of all phenomena. This quietens the analytical mind and generates the space for openness, honesty and sensitivity to function, as the natural expressions of unhindered awareness. At the same time it undermines the habit of identifying with experiences and actions, so fundamental to the deeper promise of yoga.

● BEING PRESENT TO THAT WHICH IS ACTUALLY HAPPENING (BRAHMACHARYA)

Is honoured through the expression of sensitivity, honesty, openness and generosity. It invites body and mind to act and experience directly, fully and freely as momentary, local expressions of the indivisible unity of totality. It is manifested as a vital directness in thought, feeling and action, which expresses a deep intimacy with body, mind, sprit and world. This resolves the habituated split between subject and object, self and other, body and mind into the light of clear awareness, expressing freely through its natural functions of presence, generosity, openness, honesty and sensitivity. In that light the inherent unity of body, mind and spirit, or being human, radiates spontaneously and naturally.

Index

Air Release **92**

Balance **35**
Big Toe Pose **64**
Boat **74**
Bow **59**
Bridge **57**

Camel **58**
Cat **72**
Chair Pose **9**
Child's Pose **86**
Cobra **53**
Cobra Variation II **54**
Corpse **87**
Cow **55**
Cow Pose **37**
Crane/Birdie **50**
Crocodile **63**

Dolphin **78**
Downwards-Facing dog **8**
Downwards-Facing Tree
  Headstand **83**

Eagle **15**
Extended Hand to Big Toe
  23
Extended Puppy **70**
Extended Side Angle **13**
Extended Triangle **14**

Firefly **51**
Fish **62**
Full Boat **73**

Garland **26**

Half Locust **48**
Half Moon **17**
Half Prayer Twist **29**
Half Spinal Twist **43**
Half Wheel I **24**
Half Wheel II **25**
Head-to-knee Forwards
  Bend **71**
Hero's Pose **31**
High Lunge **10**
Horse Gesture in Shoulder
  Stand **80**

Kneeling Dancer Pose **61**

Leg-Raise **85**
Lifted Lotus **40**
Locust **47**
Lord of the Dance **22**
Lotus **30**
Low Lunge **11**

Marichi I **68**
Meditation **89**
Mountain **6**
Mountain **38**

Noose **36**

Pigeon **56**
Plank **46**
Plough **81**
Prayer Twist **28**
Properous/Auspicious **34**
Propped Rabbit **91**

Reclining Big Toe **93**
Reclining Hero **90**
Reversed Corpse **88**
Revolded Side Lunge **12**
Revolved Head to Knee **45**

Scorpion **84**
Seated Forwards Bend **66**
Seated Forwards Bend **67**
Shoulder Stand **79**
Shoulder-Pressing Pose **77**
Side Plank **49**
Side-Reclining Leg Lift **75**
Side-Reclining Leg Lift II
  76
Staff **33**
Standing Forward Bend **7**
Standing Half-Forwards
  Bend **69**
Standing Split **27**
Supported Headstand **82**

Three-Legged Dog **16**
Thunderbolt **32**
Tied Lotus **41**
Tree Pose **18**
Triangle Pose **21**

Twisted Pose I **44**
Type 1 Bow Pose in Sitting
  42

Upward Bow/Wheel **60**
Upwards-Facing Dog **52**

Warrior I **19**
Warrior II **20**
Wide-Angled Seated
  Forwards Bend **39**
Wide-Legged Forwards
  Bend **65**